C-PAP Without the Hype

What Sleep Apnea Does,

Why C-PAP matters,

And how to make it work in real life.

T. L. Everheart

This book is intended for informational and educational purposes only. It is not a substitute for professional medical advice, diagnosis, or treatment. Always seek the guidance of a qualified healthcare provider with any questions regarding a medical condition or treatment. Never disregard professional medical advice or delay seeking it because of something you have read in this book.

While every effort has been made to ensure the accuracy of the information in this book, the author and publisher make no representations or warranties regarding completeness or results from the use of this information, and disclaim any liability for adverse outcomes arising from its use.

Published by The Lemon Grove

Printed in the United States of America

How to Use This Book

This book is meant to be practical, not overwhelming.

You do not need to read it cover to cover in one sitting. Some people start at the beginning to understand sleep apnea itself. Others jump straight to the chapters about CPAP, comfort, or long-term use because that is what they are dealing with right now.

Each chapter focuses on one part of the process, from diagnosis to treatment to everyday life with therapy. You can read in order, skip around, or return to sections later as questions come up.

This book is not a replacement for your medical provider, but it is meant to help you understand what they are telling you and what real-life treatment often looks like outside the office.

Use it as a reference, a guide, or simply reassurance that what you are experiencing is normal and manageable.

Dedication

This book is dedicated to everyone who had to lie awake next to me, listen to me snore, or sit there wondering if I was going to start breathing again.

Thank you for the concern, the nudges, and the patience. You were noticing something I did not fully understand yet. This book exists in part because of you.

Author's Note

This book came from a simple problem.

When I was diagnosed with sleep apnea, my doctor explained what was happening and what treatment might look like. The information was helpful, but once I got home, I realized I could not find all of it in one place.

What I found instead was scattered articles, technical explanations, or information tied to selling a specific machine, product, or method. I wanted something straightforward that explained what sleep apnea is, what treatment actually feels like, and what real progress usually looks like.

It also took me time to see results. Not days or weeks, but months. Looking back, I can see the small steps adding up, even when they did not feel dramatic in the moment. I still wish I could jump out of bed the way I used to, but the trade-off is that I no longer feel like I need a nap just to get through the day. That alone makes a difference.

This book is not meant to replace medical advice, and it does not push one single solution. It is simply meant to explain the process in clear language so you know what is happening, what to expect, and what improvement often looks like in real life.

If it helps you feel less confused, less overwhelmed, or more prepared for what comes next, then it has done its job.

T.L. Everheart

Table of Contents

Chapter One

What Sleep Apnea Is

What's Actually Happening When You Stop Breathing

Most people hear the term *sleep apnea* and think it just means snoring, tossing and turning, or maybe waking up tired. It sounds like a sleep nuisance, not a serious medical issue.

But sleep apnea isn't just noisy sleep. It's a breathing problem that happens while you're unconscious, and that makes it easy to ignore for years.

To understand sleep apnea, it helps to understand what's supposed to happen when you sleep.

What Normal Breathing During Sleep Looks Like

When you fall asleep, your body naturally relaxes. Your muscles loosen, your breathing slows, and your nervous system shifts into a more restorative mode. This is normal and healthy. Your airway; the passage that air travels through from your nose and mouth into your lungs is supposed to stay open enough for air to move freely.

For most people, it does.

But for people with obstructive sleep apnea, the airway doesn't stay open the way it should. When the muscles relax, the tongue, soft palate, or surrounding tissue can fall backward and narrow the airway. In some cases, it partially blocks airflow. In other cases, it closes off almost completely.

When that happens, breathing either becomes shallow or stops altogether.

What Happens When the Airway Closes

The moment airflow drops, oxygen levels in the blood begin to fall. Your body notices this quickly. Your brain is designed to protect breathing above almost everything else, even when you're asleep.

When oxygen drops, the brain sends an emergency signal to wake you up just enough to reopen the airway. You might snort, gasp, shift positions, or tighten the muscles in your throat. Then breathing resumes.

This awakening is usually very brief. Most people don't remember it. They don't sit up or fully wake. They just move from deeper sleep into lighter sleep for a moment and then drift off again.

But that moment matters.

Because for some people, this cycle happens over and over all night long.

Not once or twice. Sometimes dozens of times. Sometimes hundreds.

Each time breathing stops or weakens, the body experiences a small stress event. Oxygen dips. The brain alarms. Sleep gets interrupted. The cycle repeats.

From the outside, a partner might hear loud snoring, choking sounds, or pauses in breathing. From the inside, the person often just feels tired without knowing why.

Why Interrupted Sleep Matters

Sleep isn't just about being unconscious for eight hours. It's a structured biological process. During a normal night, your brain moves through different sleep stages, including light sleep, deep sleep, and REM sleep. Each stage has a job.

Deep sleep is when your body repairs tissues, strengthens your immune system, and restores energy.
REM sleep is when your brain processes memory, emotions, and learning.
Both are essential.

When apnea repeatedly interrupts breathing, your brain keeps pulling you out of those deeper stages to reopen the airway. Even if you never wake fully, you're pushed into lighter sleep again and again.

It's like trying to charge your phone overnight but unplugging it every few minutes. It technically spent all night on the charger, but it never actually finished charging.

That's why people with untreated sleep apnea can sleep for eight hours and still feel exhausted.

It's not about how long you slept.
It's about whether your body ever got the chance to fully rest.

The Body's Stress Response

Each breathing interruption also activates your body's stress system.

When oxygen drops, your body releases stress hormones like adrenaline. Your heart rate changes. Your blood pressure rises. Your nervous system shifts into alert mode so you can breathe again.

This response is helpful in the moment: It keeps you alive.

But when it happens repeatedly night after night, it puts strain on the body. Over time, this repeated stress can contribute to high blood pressure, heart problems, blood sugar issues, and chronic fatigue.

It also affects how your brain works during the day. Many people with untreated apnea experience brain fog, forgetfulness, irritability, or trouble concentrating. Some feel emotionally flat or unusually anxious. Others notice they fall asleep easily during quiet moments like watching TV, reading, or sitting in meetings.

These symptoms don't always get linked to sleep right away. People often blame stress, age, weight, work schedules, or just being busy. Sleep apnea can hide in plain sight for years.

Why Many People Don't Notice It

One of the hardest parts about sleep apnea is that it happens while you're unconscious. You don't see it. You don't remember it. You just feel the effects.

Some people only get tested because a partner notices they stop breathing. Others get tested after years of unexplained fatigue, high blood pressure, or morning headaches. Some are diagnosed during routine screenings because they fall into higher-risk groups.

By the time many people learn they have sleep apnea, the condition has often been affecting their body for a long time.

Understanding what's happening in your body is the first step toward understanding why treatment matters.

CPAP isn't just about stopping snoring.
It's about preventing this cycle of airway collapse, oxygen drops, and stress responses so your body can finally get the kind of sleep it's been missing.

For many people, hearing they have sleep apnea feels sudden, but the condition itself usually isn't. It often develops slowly, with symptoms building so gradually that they start to feel normal. Being tired becomes routine. Headaches become expected. Foggy thinking gets blamed on stress or getting older.

Understanding what sleep apnea actually is helps explain why those symptoms happen, and why treatment isn't just about sleeping better. It's about stopping a cycle that strains the body night after night.

In the next chapter, we'll look at why sleep apnea makes people feel so exhausted, even when they think they've been sleeping all night, and how those interrupted nights start to show up in everyday life.

Chapter Two

Why You Feel Exhausted Even After Sleeping

Sleeping does not always mean resting.

One of the most frustrating parts of sleep apnea is how tired people feel even after spending a full night in bed.

Many people assume exhaustion means they didn't sleep long enough. So they try going to bed earlier. They sleep in on weekends. They take naps when they can. And still, the fatigue doesn't go away.

That's because sleep apnea isn't a problem of time in bed.
It's a problem of what happens during that time.

To understand why sleep apnea makes people so exhausted, it helps to understand what sleep is supposed to do for the body — and what happens when that process keeps getting interrupted.

Sleep Isn't Just "Turning Off"

A lot of people think of sleep as a simple switch. You're awake, then you're asleep, and after enough hours you should feel rested.

In reality, sleep is a structured cycle that the brain moves through repeatedly during the night. These cycles include lighter stages of sleep, deeper restorative stages, and REM sleep, where dreaming often occurs. Each stage serves a different function, and all of them matter.

During deep sleep, the body repairs tissues, releases growth hormones, strengthens immune function, and restores physical energy. This is the phase where the body does much of its maintenance work.

REM sleep, on the other hand, is when the brain processes memory, learning, and emotions. It's important for concentration, mood regulation, and mental clarity.

A normal night of sleep cycles smoothly through these stages several times. The deeper stages become longer as the night goes on, which is why the second half of the night often feels especially restorative.

Sleep apnea disrupts this entire pattern.

How Apnea Interrupts the Sleep Cycle

When your airway collapses and breathing slows or stops, the brain senses that oxygen levels are dropping. As described in the previous chapter, it sends a signal that pulls you into lighter sleep just long enough to reopen the airway.

Even if you don't fully wake up, that interruption matters. Each time it happens, it cuts off the deeper stage you were in and forces your brain to restart the sleep cycle again.

Imagine trying to watch a movie, but every few minutes someone turns the TV off and back on. You might still technically be sitting there for two hours, but you never really get to follow the story. Sleep apnea works the same way. Your body spends hours in bed, but it never gets to stay in the stages that actually restore you.

Some people experience these interruptions dozens of times per night. Others experience them hundreds of times. The exact number depends on how severe the apnea is, but even moderate disruption can have noticeable effects.

The result is fragmented sleep. It's not always obvious in the moment, but over time the impact becomes very real.

The Brain Never Fully Powers Down

One of the key jobs of sleep is to let the brain reset. When sleep is uninterrupted, the brain reduces sensory input, processes information from the day, and prepares for the next one.

When breathing interruptions keep happening, the brain stays in a kind of half-alert mode all night. It's constantly monitoring oxygen levels and triggering brief awakenings to keep the airway open.

That means the brain never fully relaxes.

This ongoing low-level alertness is part of why people with sleep apnea often wake up feeling mentally foggy or unrefreshed. It's not just that they slept poorly. It's that their brain spent the entire night on standby instead of getting real rest.

Many people describe this feeling as waking up already tired. Others say they feel like they could fall back asleep immediately after getting out of bed. Some feel sluggish and slow to think for the first hour or more of the day.

These symptoms aren't random. They're the direct result of a brain that never got the uninterrupted rest it needed.

The Stress Hormone Effect

Another reason sleep apnea leads to exhaustion has to do with the body's stress response.

Each time breathing stops and oxygen dips, the body releases stress hormones like adrenaline and cortisol. These chemicals are designed to help you respond to danger. They raise your heart rate, increase blood pressure, and make your body more alert.

In a true emergency, this response is lifesaving.

But when it happens repeatedly during sleep, it becomes a problem. Instead of spending the night in a calm, restorative state, your body cycles through small bursts of stress over and over again.

This constant activation can leave you feeling wired but tired. Some people notice that they wake up feeling restless, tense, or anxious without knowing why. Others experience morning headaches, a racing heart, or a sense that they never fully relaxed overnight.

Over time, this stress response can also affect blood pressure, blood sugar regulation, and overall energy levels. The body isn't meant to spend the night in a repeated alarm cycle. It's meant to recover.

Why You May Not Realize How Bad It Is

One of the tricky things about sleep apnea fatigue is that it develops gradually. People don't usually wake up one day feeling dramatically worse than the day before. Instead, the tiredness builds slowly.

At first, it might feel like needing an extra cup of coffee. Then it becomes needing caffeine just to get through the morning. Later, it might feel like fighting sleep during meetings, needing naps, or losing focus more easily.

Because the change is gradual, people often adapt to it. They assume this is just what getting older feels like, or what a busy life feels like. They adjust their expectations instead of questioning their sleep.

Some people only realize how tired they've been after they start treatment and finally experience real restorative sleep again. That contrast can be eye-opening.

Daytime Symptoms That Connect Back to Nighttime Sleep

The effects of poor sleep show up in different ways for different people. Some experience overwhelming fatigue. Others notice more subtle changes.

Common daytime effects of untreated sleep apnea can include difficulty concentrating, forgetfulness, irritability, reduced patience, low motivation, or feeling emotionally drained. Some people feel unusually sensitive to stress. Others feel numb or detached.

Physical symptoms can show up too. Morning headaches, dry mouth, or sore throat can be signs of disrupted breathing. Some people notice weight changes or increased cravings, which can be linked to hormonal shifts from poor sleep.

Not everyone experiences all of these symptoms, but most people with untreated sleep apnea notice at least some of them once they know what to look for.

Why More Sleep Alone Doesn't Fix It

One of the biggest misconceptions about sleep apnea is that it can be solved by simply sleeping longer.

If the airway keeps collapsing, the problem isn't the number of hours in bed. It's the quality of those hours. Without treatment, the interruptions continue no matter how early you go to bed.

That's why people with untreated sleep apnea can sleep for nine or ten hours and still feel exhausted. The body never got the uninterrupted deep sleep it needed to recharge.

Treatment works not because it makes you sleep longer, but because it helps restore the structure of normal sleep cycles. When breathing stays steady, the brain can stay in deeper sleep stages for longer periods. Over time, that allows the body to recover in ways it hasn't been able to.

What Many People Notice After Treatment Begins

Not everyone feels dramatically better on the first night of treatment, but many people do notice gradual changes once their sleep becomes more stable.

Some report clearer thinking in the morning. Others feel less irritable or more patient during the day. Energy levels often improve slowly rather than all at once. For people who have lived with untreated apnea for years, the change can feel subtle at first, then increasingly noticeable.

It's important to understand that improvement can take time. The body may need weeks or months of better sleep to fully recover from long-term disruption. But restoring breathing during sleep is the first step in allowing that recovery to happen.

Sleep apnea doesn't just make you tired. It prevents your body from doing the work it's supposed to do overnight. Treatment isn't about perfection or loving the machine. It's about giving your brain and body a chance to finally rest the way they're meant to.

Chapter Three

The Health Effects People Don't Always Connect to Sleep

By the time many people are diagnosed with sleep apnea, they've already been living with its effects for years. The problem is that those effects rarely show up in a way that clearly points back to sleep.

Instead, they appear as everyday health issues that seem unrelated at first. High blood pressure. Brain fog. Mood changes. Weight struggles. Headaches. Fatigue that doesn't make sense. Each symptom gets treated on its own, but the underlying cause often goes unnoticed.

Sleep apnea doesn't just make you tired. It affects multiple systems in the body, and it does it slowly enough that people often adjust to the changes without realizing what's happening.

The Oxygen Problem

At the core of sleep apnea is one simple issue: repeated drops in oxygen.

Every time the airway collapses, airflow decreases or stops. Oxygen levels in the blood fall, sometimes only slightly, sometimes more significantly. Each drop triggers the brain's alarm system, forcing the body to wake just enough to reopen the airway.

These repeated oxygen dips are stressful for the body. While one or two short drops wouldn't cause lasting harm, hundreds of them every night over months or years can create a pattern of strain.

The body isn't built to function well when oxygen supply keeps fluctuating. Cells rely on steady oxygen levels to produce energy, repair tissue, and maintain normal function. When that supply is inconsistent, the body compensates by increasing stress signals, raising blood pressure, and altering hormone patterns.

These adjustments help in the short term, but over time they contribute to broader health problems.

The Heart and Blood Pressure Connection

One of the strongest links researchers have found is between sleep apnea and cardiovascular health.

When breathing stops during sleep, the body releases stress hormones that cause blood vessels to tighten and blood pressure to rise. Heart rate may increase or fluctuate. These changes are meant to protect oxygen delivery, but when they happen repeatedly, they put extra workload on the heart and circulation.

Many people with untreated sleep apnea develop high blood pressure that's difficult to control with medication alone. Some experience irregular heart rhythms. Others are at increased risk for heart disease or stroke over time.

The connection isn't always obvious to patients, because heart problems develop gradually. A person may simply be told they have hypertension or need medication, without realizing their sleep could be part of the reason.

Treating sleep apnea doesn't replace other medical treatment, but it often plays an important role in stabilizing these systems.

The Brain and Cognitive Effects

Sleep apnea also affects how the brain functions during the day.

When sleep is repeatedly interrupted and oxygen dips occur, the brain doesn't get the consistent restorative time it needs. Over time, this can affect memory, concentration, and mental sharpness.

People often describe this as brain fog. They may forget conversations, misplace things, struggle to focus on tasks, or feel slower in their thinking than they used to. Some notice they have trouble finding words or keeping track of details.

These changes can be subtle at first. Many people assume they're just stressed, aging, or overwhelmed. But disrupted sleep can have a measurable impact on cognitive performance.

Mood is affected too. Poor sleep can increase irritability, reduce patience, and make emotional regulation harder. Anxiety and depression often worsen when sleep quality declines. In some cases, people feel emotionally flat or disconnected without understanding why.

The brain relies on sleep to reset itself. When that reset keeps getting interrupted, the effects show up during the day.

Hormones, Weight, and Metabolism

Sleep apnea can also influence hormones that regulate hunger, energy use, and metabolism.

When sleep is disrupted, the balance of hormones like leptin and ghrelin shifts. These hormones help control appetite and fullness. When they're out of balance, people may feel hungrier, crave higher-calorie foods, or have difficulty feeling satisfied after eating.

Poor sleep can also reduce insulin sensitivity, making it harder for the body to regulate blood sugar efficiently. Over time, this can contribute to weight gain and metabolic issues.

This creates a frustrating cycle. Weight gain can increase the severity of sleep apnea by adding pressure around the airway. At the same time, untreated apnea can make weight harder to manage because of hormonal shifts and fatigue.

Understanding this cycle can help explain why lifestyle changes alone sometimes don't produce the expected results until sleep quality improves.

Morning Symptoms That Get Overlooked

Some effects of sleep apnea show up immediately after waking, but they're often brushed off as normal.

Morning headaches are common, especially dull headaches that fade after an hour or two. These can be related to oxygen fluctuations or poor sleep quality.

Dry mouth or sore throat can result from breathing through the mouth or air leaks during sleep.

Some people wake feeling groggy or disoriented, needing extra time to fully wake up. Others feel like they never really slept at all, even if they were in bed for hours.

Because these symptoms fade during the day, they often don't get reported to doctors unless someone asks specifically.

Why It Often Takes So Long to Connect the Dots

One reason sleep apnea goes undiagnosed for so long is that its symptoms don't always look dramatic. People keep functioning. They go to work, take care of responsibilities, and push through fatigue because that's what they've always done.

Over time, the body adapts to running on poor sleep. What once felt abnormal starts to feel routine. By the time someone gets evaluated, they may not even remember what well-rested felt like.

It's also common for people to think of sleep as separate from the rest of their health. They don't always realize how deeply it affects blood pressure, mood, metabolism, and mental clarity.

Understanding these connections can help explain why treatment matters. CPAP isn't just about reducing snoring or improving comfort at night. It's about stabilizing breathing so the body can stop compensating for oxygen drops and interrupted sleep.

For many people, recognizing how much sleep apnea affects their health is the turning point that makes treatment feel worthwhile instead of optional.

Chapter Four

How Sleep Apnea Develops Over Time

For some people, sleep apnea seems to appear suddenly. One day they're told they snore loudly or stop breathing at night, and the diagnosis feels unexpected. In reality, sleep apnea usually doesn't begin overnight. It tends to develop gradually, often over years, as small changes in the body and sleep patterns add up.

Understanding how sleep apnea develops helps explain why so many people live with it for a long time before realizing what's happening.

The Role of the Airway

At its core, obstructive sleep apnea is a mechanical issue. It happens when the airway becomes narrow enough during sleep that airflow is reduced or blocked.

Everyone's airway is slightly different. Some people naturally have a wider, more stable airway. Others have a narrower airway due to genetics, jaw structure, nasal anatomy, or soft tissue distribution. These differences may not cause noticeable problems during the day, but they can matter once the body relaxes during sleep.

As the muscles relax, the airway naturally becomes a little smaller. For people whose airway is already borderline narrow, that relaxation can be enough to cause repeated collapse.

For some individuals, this vulnerability has been present since childhood or early adulthood, even if symptoms weren't obvious at first.

Gradual Changes Over Time

For many people, sleep apnea develops as a result of changes that happen slowly over time.

Weight gain is one of the most well-known contributors. Extra tissue around the neck and airway can increase the likelihood of collapse during sleep. Even modest changes in weight can affect airway stability, especially if fat distribution occurs around the throat.

But weight isn't the only factor.

Aging also plays a role. As we get older, muscle tone throughout the body changes, including in the throat. The tissues that help keep the airway open may become less firm, making collapse more likely during sleep.

Hormonal shifts can contribute as well. For example, some women develop sleep apnea after menopause, when hormonal changes affect muscle tone and fat distribution. This can happen even in women who never had symptoms earlier in life.

Nasal congestion, chronic sinus issues, or structural changes in the nose can also make airflow more difficult, increasing the likelihood that the body will compensate by mouth breathing during sleep. This can further affect airway stability.

Individually, these changes may seem small. Together, they can shift the airway from stable to vulnerable.

Why Symptoms Often Start Subtly

One reason sleep apnea is often missed is that it rarely begins dramatically. Instead, symptoms tend to creep in slowly.

Snoring might start quietly and become louder over time. Morning fatigue may appear occasionally before becoming more consistent. A person might notice they wake up more often, or that they don't feel as refreshed in the morning as they used to.

Because the changes are gradual, they're easy to dismiss. People attribute them to stress, work schedules, aging, or lifestyle changes. By the time the symptoms are strong enough to prompt a sleep study, the condition may have been developing for years.

Some people are diagnosed only after a partner notices breathing pauses at night. Others are referred for testing because of persistent fatigue, high blood pressure, or unexplained headaches. Occasionally, the diagnosis comes during an evaluation for something else entirely.

The slow progression of sleep apnea is one reason it's so common and yet so often overlooked.

Lifelong vs. Later-Onset Apnea

Not everyone develops sleep apnea the same way. For some people, the tendency toward airway collapse has been present for much of their life. They may have always snored, even as children or young adults, but the condition wasn't recognized as a medical issue.

For others, sleep apnea truly does develop later. Weight changes, hormonal shifts, aging, or medical conditions can push the airway from stable to unstable over time.

Understanding which pattern fits your experience can help explain why symptoms appeared when they did. It also helps reinforce that sleep apnea isn't a personal failure or something caused by a single choice. It's usually the result of multiple factors interacting over time.

Why People Often Don't Seek Help Right Away

Because sleep apnea develops gradually and symptoms can be explained away, many people delay getting evaluated. Fatigue becomes something they work around rather than something they question. Snoring becomes a joke instead of a warning sign.

Some people avoid testing because they worry about being told they need CPAP. Others assume their symptoms aren't serious enough to matter. Some simply don't realize sleep apnea can affect so many aspects of health.

By the time they do get tested, many people are surprised at how long the condition may have been affecting them.

Understanding the Bigger Picture

Recognizing how sleep apnea develops can make the diagnosis feel less mysterious. It helps explain why treatment isn't just about solving a recent problem. It's about addressing a process that may have been building quietly for years.

In the next chapter, we'll look more closely at the specific risk factors that make some people more likely to develop sleep apnea than others, and why anatomy, weight, and other physical factors all play a role.

Chapter Five

Weight, Anatomy, and Why Some People Are More at Risk

When people hear about sleep apnea, one of the first things they often hear is that it's linked to weight. That connection is real, but it's also incomplete. Sleep apnea is influenced by a combination of physical factors, and weight is only one piece of a larger picture.

Understanding these factors can help explain why some people develop sleep apnea while others don't, even when their lifestyles look similar.

The Airway Is a Physical Space

At its simplest level, breathing depends on having enough open space in the airway for air to move in and out of the lungs. Anything that narrows that space or makes it less stable during sleep can increase the risk of obstruction.

The shape of your jaw, the position of your tongue, the size of your tonsils, and the structure of your nasal passages all affect how easily air flows. These features are largely determined by genetics. Some people are born with wider airways that stay open easily. Others naturally have narrower airways that are more likely to collapse when muscles relax during sleep.

This means that two people with the same body weight can have very different levels of risk depending on their anatomy.

How Weight Affects the Airway

Weight plays a role because fat distribution around the neck and throat can reduce the available airway space. Extra tissue in this area can make the airway more likely to narrow or collapse when the body relaxes during sleep.

Even modest weight gain can influence this. It doesn't always take a large change to affect airway stability, especially for someone whose airway was already somewhat narrow to begin with.

Weight can also affect breathing mechanics more broadly. Increased abdominal weight can reduce lung expansion when lying down, which may contribute to changes in breathing patterns during sleep.

But it's important to remember that weight alone doesn't determine whether someone will develop sleep apnea. Some people at higher weights don't have apnea at all, while others at lower weights do.

Framing sleep apnea only as a "weight problem" can cause people to overlook other important factors and delay getting evaluated when symptoms appear.

Jaw Structure and Facial Anatomy

The shape of the lower jaw and the position of the tongue can also influence airway stability.

People with a smaller or more recessed jaw may have less room in the back of the throat for the tongue and soft tissues. When those tissues relax during sleep, they can crowd the airway more easily.

Similarly, a naturally larger tongue or thicker soft palate can contribute to airway narrowing. These features aren't visible from the outside, which is one reason sleep apnea risk isn't always obvious based on appearance alone.

Dental and orthodontic history sometimes provides clues. People who had significant crowding, braces, or certain bite patterns may have structural features that affect airway space, although not everyone with these traits develops apnea.

Nasal and Sinus Factors

Breathing comfortably through the nose helps keep airflow steady and the airway stable. Chronic nasal congestion, sinus issues, or structural differences like a deviated septum can make nasal breathing harder.

When the nose is blocked, people often compensate by breathing through the mouth. Mouth breathing can change how the jaw and tongue position themselves during sleep, which may increase the chance of airway collapse.

These issues don't always cause sleep apnea on their own, but they can contribute to the overall picture.

Neck Size and Fat Distribution

Where the body stores fat can matter as much as how much is present.

Some people tend to store more fat around the neck and upper airway, which can increase pressure on the throat during sleep. Others store fat more around the hips or abdomen, which may have less direct effect on airway structure.

Neck circumference is sometimes used as one rough indicator of apnea risk, but it's not a perfect measure. It's simply one piece of information that can suggest whether airway crowding might be contributing to symptoms.

Why Blame Doesn't Help

Because weight is often mentioned in discussions of sleep apnea, some people assume the condition is entirely preventable or the result of personal choices. That assumption can create unnecessary guilt or shame, which doesn't help anyone get treated.

In reality, sleep apnea is usually the result of multiple overlapping factors. Genetics, anatomy, aging, hormones, nasal structure, and weight can all play roles. Many of these are outside a person's direct control.

Understanding this can make it easier to approach treatment as a medical issue rather than a personal failure. The goal isn't to assign blame. It's to recognize what's happening and address it in a way that improves health and quality of life.

Why Risk Factors Matter

Knowing the factors that increase risk helps explain why doctors may recommend testing even when symptoms seem mild. It also helps explain why sleep apnea can affect people at many different body sizes and ages.

In the next chapter, we'll look more closely at how sleep apnea can present differently in men and women, and why women are often diagnosed later even when symptoms are present.

Chapter Six

How Sleep Apnea Is Diagnosed

Most people don't wake up one morning knowing they have sleep apnea.
They just know something feels off.

They wake up tired. They fall asleep in the afternoon. Their partner complains about snoring or pauses in breathing. They start wondering if this is just aging… stress… or something else.

Diagnosis usually begins with that quiet realization: *This isn't normal.*

Step One: Talking to a Provider

Diagnosis often starts with a primary care visit. A provider may ask questions like:

- Do you snore loudly?
  - Has anyone seen you stop breathing during sleep?
- Do you wake up choking or gasping?
- Are you tired during the day?
- Do you wake with headaches?
- Do you have high blood pressure?

None of these questions alone confirm apnea. But together, they help determine whether testing makes sense.

Many providers also use short screening tools like the **STOP-BANG questionnaire**, which looks at snoring, tiredness, blood pressure, body size, age, and gender risk factors.

If screening suggests possible apnea, the next step is sleep testing.

Step Two: Sleep Studies

Sleep apnea is diagnosed using a sleep study. This measures breathing, oxygen levels, heart rate, and sleep patterns overnight.

There are two main types.

In-Lab Sleep Study (Polysomnography)

This is the traditional, most detailed option.

You spend the night in a sleep center while sensors measure:

- Brain waves (sleep stages)
- Breathing patterns
- Oxygen levels

- Heart rate
- Leg movements
- Body position
- Airflow through nose and mouth

It sounds intimidating, but most people are surprised how manageable it is.
You sleep in a quiet room, not a hospital ward, and the goal is simply to capture a typical night of sleep.

In-lab studies are often recommended when:

- Symptoms are severe
- Other sleep disorders are suspected
- Prior tests were unclear
- Medical conditions complicate the picture

Home Sleep Apnea Testing

Many people now qualify for home testing.

This involves wearing a small monitor overnight that tracks:

- Breathing effort
- Oxygen levels
- Airflow

- Sometimes heart rate

It's simpler and more comfortable than lab testing, but it gathers less data.

Home studies work well for people with a high suspicion of obstructive sleep apnea and no major complicating conditions.

If a home study is unclear or negative but symptoms remain strong, a lab study may still be needed.

What the Results Actually Show

Sleep study results focus on something called the ***AHI-Apnea-Hypopnea Index***.

This number shows how many breathing interruptions happen per hour.

- **5–15 events/hour** → Mild apnea
- **15–30 events/hour** → Moderate apnea
- **30+ events/hour** → Severe apnea

But the number alone doesn't tell the whole story.

Oxygen drops, heart rate changes, and sleep fragmentation all matter too.
Some people with moderate numbers feel terrible.
Others with severe apnea didn't realize how bad they felt until treatment started.

Diagnosis is about the full picture, not just a single score.

Why Diagnosis Matters

Some people hesitate to get tested because they worry it will lead to equipment, machines, or major life changes.

But testing doesn't force treatment.
It just gives you information.

Knowing what's happening during sleep helps explain symptoms that may have felt random or unrelated.

For many people, diagnosis is the moment things finally start to make sense.

Fatigue.
Brain fog.
Morning headaches.

Mood changes.
Blood pressure issues.

Instead of guessing, you finally know what your body has been dealing with. And once you know, you can decide what to do next.

Chapter Seven

What Happens After Diagnosis

Getting diagnosed with sleep apnea can feel like a strange mix of relief and worry.

Relief, because there is finally an explanation for what's been happening.
Worry, because now there's a decision to make about treatment.

Some people imagine diagnosis means they'll immediately be handed a machine and told they have no choice.
In reality, the process is usually more gradual and more collaborative than that.

Diagnosis gives you information.
Treatment decisions come next.

Understanding the Recommendation

After your sleep study is reviewed, a provider will go over the results with you.

They'll explain:

- How often breathing stopped
- How low oxygen levels dropped
- How fragmented your sleep was

- Whether apnea was mild, moderate, or severe

From there, they'll recommend treatment options.

For most people with moderate to severe obstructive sleep apnea, CPAP therapy is the first-line treatment because it is the most effective way to keep the airway open.

But that doesn't mean it's the only option, and it doesn't mean you're locked into anything permanently.

Treatment is about improving sleep and health, not forcing a specific device.

The First CPAP Conversation

For many people, this is the moment anxiety kicks in.

They picture bulky hospital machines, noisy equipment, or feeling trapped behind a mask.That image is outdated.

Modern CPAP machines are small, quiet, and designed for home use.

Masks come in multiple styles and sizes, and fitting is part of the process, not an afterthought.

At this stage, you're usually referred to a durable medical equipment provider (DME).
They help with:

- Machine setup
- Mask fitting
- Pressure settings
- Insurance paperwork
- Education on how to use the equipment

This isn't a one-time handoff.
There's usually follow-up, adjustments, and troubleshooting as you get used to therapy.

What If You're Not Ready for CPAP Yet?

Some people need time to process the diagnosis before starting treatment.
Others want to explore alternatives first.

Depending on severity and anatomy, options may include:

- Oral appliance therapy (custom dental device)

- Positional therapy (training to avoid back sleeping)
- Weight management strategies
- Nasal treatment for congestion or obstruction
- Surgery in select cases

CPAP remains the most reliable treatment for moderate to severe apnea, but it's not the only conversation. The goal is to find something that works for your body and your life.

Why Treatment Is Worth Considering

Untreated sleep apnea doesn't just mean snoring or fatigue.
It keeps the body in a cycle of stress every night.

When breathing repeatedly stops, the brain sends emergency signals that raise heart rate and blood pressure.
Over time, this contributes to cardiovascular strain, insulin resistance, and persistent exhaustion.

Treatment isn't about perfection.
It's about reducing that nightly stress load on the body.

Many people don't realize how poorly they were sleeping until treatment begins.
Some notice changes within days.
Others improve gradually over weeks.

Better sleep often shows up as:

- More stable energy
- Fewer morning headaches
- Improved mood
- Clearer thinking
- Less daytime sleepiness

These changes can be subtle at first, but they build over time.

The Adjustment Phase

No matter which treatment path you choose, there's usually an adjustment period.

This is normal.

Learning to sleep with equipment, changing habits, or adapting to new routines takes time.
It doesn't mean treatment isn't working , it means your body and brain are learning something new.

Most successful long-term users weren't instantly comfortable.
They improved through small adjustments, troubleshooting, and persistence.

Progress matters more than perfection.

Moving Forward

Diagnosis isn't the end of the process.
It's the beginning of understanding what your body needs.

Treatment decisions don't have to happen all at once.
You can ask questions, try options, make adjustments, and take this step by step.

The goal isn't to force you into a device.
The goal is to help you sleep in a way that supports your health, energy, and daily life.

And once treatment starts, the next question naturally becomes: *What is CPAP actually like to use?*

Chapter Eight

Starting CPAP: What the First Nights Are Really Like

The first night using CPAP is rarely magical.

For some people, it's fine.For most, it's an adjustment.

You're sleeping with something new on your face, breathing with assisted airflow, and paying attention to sleep in a way you never have before. That alone can feel strange.

Knowing what's normal makes the process much easier.

It May Feel Weird at First

CPAP works by gently pushing air into your airway so it stays open during sleep. That airflow isn't dangerous or forceful, but it can feel unfamiliar in the beginning.

Some people describe it as:

- Feeling like there's too much air
- Feeling like they can't exhale normally
- Feeling hyper-aware of their breathing
- Worrying the mask will move or leak

This usually improves within a few nights as your brain stops treating the mask like a problem.

Modern machines also have comfort features like ramp settings and exhale relief that make this transition easier.

Your Sleep Might Not Be Perfect Right Away

This part surprises people.

You may actually sleep worse the first few nights.

Not because CPAP is harmful, but because anything new can disrupt sleep temporarily.

You might:

- Wake up adjusting the mask
- Notice the airflow
- Feel unsure how to move in bed
- Be more aware of your body than usual

That doesn't mean therapy isn't working.
It means your brain is learning a new normal.

Your Nose, Mouth, or Skin Might Get Irritated

This is extremely common and very fixable.

Depending on the mask style, you may notice:

- A sore nose bridge
- Tender nostrils from nasal pillows
- Dry nose or mouth
- Skin irritation where the mask touches
- Mild pressure marks in the morning

Your nose may be sore at first, especially with nasal masks or nasal pillow styles that sit directly against the nostrils. This doesn't mean the mask is wrong, but it may need adjusting, resizing, or switching styles.

Small changes often solve this quickly:

- Loosening straps slightly
- Using mask liners or cushions
- Adjusting humidity settings
- Trying a different mask type
- Using a small amount of approved skin barrier product

Discomfort early on is common. Ongoing pain is not something you just “have to live with.” There are almost always fixes.

Air Leaks Happen - and They’re Not a Failure

Another early frustration is mask leaks.

You might feel air blowing toward your eyes or hear a soft whooshing sound.
This doesn’t mean you’re doing something wrong.

Masks shift as you move during sleep, and finding the right fit sometimes takes a few adjustments.

Most leaks are solved by:

- Minor strap adjustments
- Repositioning the mask while lying down
- Trying a different size cushion
- Switching mask styles if needed

This is part of the normal learning curve, not a sign you can’t use CPAP.

You Might Not Feel Better Immediately

Some people wake up after one night feeling dramatically better.
Most don't.

Sleep recovery takes time.

Your body may need days or weeks of consistent sleep before you notice real changes in energy, mood, or clarity. That doesn't mean nothing is happening, it means your system is catching up on something it's been missing for years.

The Goal of the First Nights

The goal isn't perfect sleep.

The goal is simply getting used to the machine.

Even a few hours of use counts as progress.
Your brain learns through repetition, not perfection.

Most long-term successful users didn't love CPAP on night one.
They improved by troubleshooting, adjusting, and giving themselves time.

What Comes Next

Once the first nights pass, the questions shift from: *"Can I tolerate this?* "to *"How do I make this comfortable long-term?"*

That's where small adjustments, habit changes, and troubleshooting make the biggest difference.

Chapter Nine

Making CPAP Comfortable: Masks, Humidity, and Fixing Common Problems

Most people who succeed with CPAP don't succeed because it felt perfect right away. They succeed because they learned how to adjust it.

CPAP comfort isn't about luck. It's about fit, setup, and small changes that make a big difference over time.

This chapter walks through the most common issues people run into - and what actually helps.

Finding the Right Mask Matters More Than the Machine

If CPAP feels uncomfortable, the mask is usually the reason.

There isn't one standard mask. There are several styles, and comfort depends heavily on anatomy, sleep position, and personal preference.

The main types include:

Nasal pillows
These sit directly at the nostrils and are the smallest option.
They work well for people who feel claustrophobic with larger masks or who sleep on their side.

Nasal masks

These cover the nose only and are one of the most common styles.
They balance stability and minimal coverage.

Full-face masks

These cover both the nose and mouth.
They're often used if you breathe through your mouth during sleep or have nasal obstruction.

No single mask is "best."
The best mask is the one you can sleep in consistently.

If a mask hurts, leaks constantly, or feels impossible to tolerate, it's not a failure — it's feedback. Adjusting mask style is part of the process, not a last resort.

Why Fit Is More Important Than Tightness

A common mistake is pulling the straps tighter to stop leaks. That often makes things worse.

Masks are designed to seal using airflow and cushion design, not pressure. Over-tightening can cause:

- Skin irritation
- Nose soreness
- Pressure marks
- Worse leaks from distorted cushions

A properly fitted mask should feel secure but not tight. If it leaves deep marks or causes pain, it usually needs adjustment rather than more pressure.

Reducing Face Marks, Lines, and Skin Irritation

One of the most common complaints people have about CPAP isn't the airflow.

It's the marks.

You might wake up with strap lines on your cheeks, pressure spots on your nose, or indents along your jaw. This is normal in the beginning, especially while your mask fit is still being adjusted.

But there are several simple ways to reduce this.

Mask liners create a barrier between your skin and the cushion, reducing pressure and friction.

Soft strap covers, often fleece, fabric, or silk-style material, wrap around the headgear and prevent the straps from digging into your face overnight.

Fabric or silk-style hose covers can help too. If the tubing rests along your cheek or jaw, it can leave lines or cause irritation. A soft cover makes the hose less noticeable, quieter against bedding, and less likely to leave marks.

Other small changes help:

- Loosening straps slightly if they're overtightened
- Adjusting mask position while lying in your normal sleep position
- Washing your face before bed so oils don't break the seal and force tighter straps
- Replacing cushions when they stiffen or flatten

For most people, early lines fade within an hour or two after waking. If marks last longer or feel painful, the mask probably needs adjusting rather than tightening.

Comfort matters, you're more likely to stay consistent if your face isn't paying the price every morning.

Humidity Settings Can Change Everything

Dryness is one of the most common reasons people struggle with CPAP.

Airflow without enough humidity can lead to:

- Dry nose
- Dry mouth
- Nosebleeds
- Sinus irritation
- Congestion

Most CPAP machines include adjustable humidifiers. Increasing humidity often improves comfort dramatically.

But more isn't always better.Too much humidity can cause:

- Condensation in the tubing ("rainout")
- Gurgling sounds
- Water collecting in the mask

The right setting is the one that keeps your airway comfortable without moisture buildup. Small adjustments over a few nights usually find the balance.

Dealing With Pressure Discomfort

Some people feel like the pressure is too strong, especially when trying to fall asleep.

Modern machines often include comfort features like:

- ***Ramp settings*** that start at lower pressure and increase gradually
- ***Exhale relief*** that reduces pressure when breathing out
- ***Auto-adjusting pressure modes*** that respond to breathing events

If pressure feels overwhelming, it doesn't mean CPAP won't work for you. It usually means settings need fine-tuning.

This is something providers or equipment teams can adjust- you don't have to troubleshoot alone.

Handling Mask Leaks Without Frustration

Leaks happen to almost everyone at some point. Instead of treating leaks as a failure, it helps to treat them as information.

Leaks often happen because:

- The cushion size isn't right
- The mask shifts when you change position
- The straps are too tight or too loose
- The mask was fitted sitting up instead of lying down

Adjustments that help:

- Fit the mask while lying in sleep position
- Re-seat the cushion once airflow starts
- Replace cushions periodically as they wear out
- Try a different mask style if leaks persist

Leaks are usually solved through small adjustments rather than major changes.

Yes… You're Sleeping With Equipment Now

There's another adjustment people don't always talk about. Using CPAP makes it visible that you're sleeping.

There's tubing. There's a mask. There's a machine beside the bed. At first, this can feel vulnerable, especially if you share a room or have a partner.

Some people worry they look strange.
Some feel self-conscious.
Some feel like it announces, *"I have a medical issue."*

That reaction is normal.

But most partners adjust quickly, and many actually sleep better once snoring and breathing pauses improve. For a lot of couples, CPAP improves sleep for both people.

If the visibility bothers you, small changes can help:

- Positioning the machine lower or behind the bed

- Using a hose holder to reduce tubing across the pillow
- Choosing a smaller mask style if medically appropriate
- Giving yourself time to get used to it

CPAP doesn't make you look sick.
It makes you look like someone who's taking care of their health.

And once better sleep starts showing up in your energy and mood, most people stop thinking about the equipment at all.

What Comes Next

Once comfort improves, CPAP starts becoming routine instead of something you think about constantly.

That's when people begin noticing the bigger changes, better energy, clearer thinking, and more stable sleep.

But before that happens, many people run into one last major obstacle: ***sticking with it long enough to see results.***

Chapter Ten

Why People Quit CPAP

(and How to Stick *with* It)

CPAP works.

That's not really debated medically.
What *is* debated in real life is whether people actually keep using it.

A lot of people stop within the first few months. Not because it doesn't help, but because the adjustment phase is harder than they expected.

Understanding why people quit makes it much easier not to.

Reason One: Expecting Instant Results

One of the biggest reasons people give up is simple disappointment.

They try CPAP for a few nights and think:
I don't feel dramatically different. Maybe this isn't worth it.

Sleep recovery doesn't always happen overnight.

Your body may have been running on fragmented sleep for years. It takes time for energy, focus, and mood to stabilize. Some people notice change in days. Others notice it gradually over weeks.

CPAP isn't a switch. It's a process.

Reason Two: Early Discomfort Feels Like Failure

The first weeks can include:

- Mask adjustments
- Minor leaks
- Learning humidity settings
- Getting used to airflow
- Figuring out how to move in bed

Some people interpret this as proof CPAP isn't for them.

In reality, this phase is normal.
Most long-term users went through it.

CPAP success isn't about finding perfection immediately.
It's about solving small problems until the system works for you.

Reason Three: Feeling Self-Conscious

Some people don't talk about this, but it matters.

Sleeping with equipment can feel vulnerable. You might worry how you look to a partner. You might feel like the machine labels you as "sick." You might just hate that it's visible.

That emotional reaction is real, and it fades faster than people expect.

Once better sleep kicks in, most people stop thinking about how they look and start caring more about how they feel.

And most partners are far more relieved by quiet breathing than bothered by a mask.

Reason Four: Thinking It Has to Be All or Nothing

Another trap is believing CPAP only counts if you use it perfectly every night for the full night.

That mindset makes people quit the moment they have a rough night.

Progress counts.

Even partial use helps your body adjust.
Even a few hours helps your brain learn the routine.
Consistency builds gradually.

The goal is improvement, not perfection.

Reason Five: Nobody Told You It Was a Learning Curve

A lot of people are handed a machine with basic instructions and little follow-up.

They assume if it feels awkward, they're doing something wrong.

But CPAP is a skill.
You learn it the same way you learn anything new, through repetition, small adjustments, and time.

The difference between people who quit and people who succeed usually isn't tolerance.

It's persistence.

How People Actually Stick With CPAP

People who stay consistent usually do a few things differently:

They ***expect an adjustment period***, instead of hoping for instant comfort.

They ***treat problems as fixable***, not as proof CPAP won't work.

They ***ask for mask or setting changes*** instead of silently struggling.

They ***focus on small wins***, like wearing it longer than the night before.

And most importantly, they ***connect the machine to how they want to feel***, not just to the diagnosis.

Better sleep.
More energy.
Fewer headaches.
Lower stress on the body.

That's the real goal.

What Happens When People Stick With It

For many people, CPAP eventually stops feeling like medical equipment.

It becomes routine.

You put it on, fall asleep, and don't think about it much. The machine fades into the background, and what stays noticeable is how you feel during the day.

That's when CPAP shifts from something you *have* to use…to something you don't want to sleep without.

What Comes Next

Once you understand why people quit, and how to get past that stage, the next question becomes: *What if CPAP still isn't the right solution for someone?*

Because while CPAP works for many people, it's not the only path.

Chapter Eleven

Alternatives to CPAP: What Other Options Exist

CPAP is the most effective treatment for moderate to severe obstructive sleep apnea. *But it's not the only option.*

Some people can't tolerate CPAP. Some improve enough with other strategies that they don't need it. Some use a combination of approaches depending on their anatomy and severity.

The goal isn't to force one treatment. The goal is to keep the airway open during sleep in a way that actually works for your body.

Oral Appliance Therapy (Dental Devices)

One of the most common alternatives to CPAP is an oral appliance.

This is a custom device made by a dentist trained in sleep medicine. It looks similar to a mouthguard and works by gently moving the lower jaw forward during sleep.

This forward position helps keep the airway from collapsing. Oral appliances are often recommended for:

- Mild to moderate sleep apnea

- People who cannot tolerate CPAP
- People who travel frequently and want a simpler option
- People whose airway collapse is strongly jaw-related

They're smaller, quieter, and easier to transport than CPAP. But they aren't perfect.

They can cause:

- Jaw soreness
- Tooth movement over time
- Bite changes if not monitored
- Less consistent airway support in severe apnea

For the right patient, though, they can be very effective and far easier to stick with.

Positional Therapy

Some people only have apnea when they sleep on their back.

In these cases, positional therapy may help reduce symptoms.

This involves training the body to sleep on the side instead of the back.
There are devices, wearable sensors, and even specialized pillows that gently discourage back-sleeping.

Positional therapy works best when:

- Apnea is mild
- Events are strongly position-dependent
- No major anatomical obstruction exists

For moderate or severe apnea, positional therapy alone usually isn't enough, but it can still be helpful combined with other treatments.

Weight Changes and Metabolic Factors

Weight loss can reduce apnea severity in some people, especially if excess tissue around the neck contributes to airway narrowing.

But this isn't a guaranteed cure.

Some people lose significant weight and still have apnea. Others improve dramatically.

Weight affects apnea risk, but it's only one factor among many, including jaw shape, tongue position, airway size, and muscle tone.

Weight-related treatment should be viewed as one piece of management, not the sole solution.

Nasal and Airway Treatment

If nasal obstruction is part of the problem, treating it can improve breathing during sleep and sometimes improve tolerance of other treatments.

This might include:

- Treating allergies or chronic inflammation
- Addressing a deviated septum
- Reducing nasal turbinate swelling
- Managing chronic sinus issues

Fixing nasal airflow doesn't always eliminate apnea, but it can make other treatments more effective and comfortable.

Surgical Options

Surgery is usually considered when other treatments fail or when anatomy strongly suggests a structural solution.

Different procedures target different parts of the airway.

Examples include:

- Removing excess soft tissue in the throat
- Correcting jaw positioning
- Nasal reconstruction procedures
- Tongue-base reduction in select cases

One of the newer surgical approaches involves an implanted nerve stimulator that helps keep airway muscles active during sleep.

Surgery can be helpful for carefully selected patients, but it isn't a guaranteed cure. Results vary widely depending on anatomy and severity.

Because of that, surgery is usually considered after conservative treatments have been explored.

Combination Approaches

For many people, the best solution isn't one single treatment. It's a combination.

Examples include:

- CPAP plus nasal treatment
- Oral appliance plus positional therapy
- Weight loss plus CPAP at lower pressure
- Surgery followed by CPAP or dental therapy

Sleep apnea management is often about layering strategies until breathing stays stable through the night.

Choosing the Right Path

There isn't one "correct" treatment for everyone.

The right approach depends on:

- Apnea severity

- Airway anatomy
- Lifestyle and sleep habits
- Medical conditions
- Personal tolerance of equipment

The most effective treatment is the one that keeps your airway open **and** that you can actually maintain long term.

A perfect solution that you won't use doesn't help. A practical solution you can stick with usually does.

What Comes Next

Once treatment is working, whether CPAP or something else, people usually begin noticing gradual changes.

Better energy.
Clearer thinking.
More stable sleep.
Sometimes even changes in blood pressure or metabolism.

That leads into the next question: *What actually improves when sleep apnea is treated consistently?*

Chapter Twelve

What Changes When You Finally Sleep Well

People often expect sleep apnea treatment to create one dramatic change.

They expect to wake up after a single night feeling like a completely different person.

Sometimes that happens.

More often, improvement shows up slowly, in ways you might not notice all at once.

Sleep recovery isn't just about feeling less tired. It affects the entire body and mind.

Energy Improves - But Usually Gradually

For many people, the first change is subtle.

You may not wake up feeling amazing.
But you might notice:

- You don't hit snooze as many times
- You stay awake through the afternoon
- You don't feel like you need a nap every day
- Evening exhaustion isn't as intense

This is your body catching up on restorative sleep it hasn't had in years.

It builds overtime rather than flipping on overnight.

Your Brain Starts Working Differently

Sleep apnea affects concentration, memory, and reaction time more than people realize.

When breathing repeatedly stops at night, the brain never fully settles into deep sleep. That fragmentation affects attention, mood, and cognitive clarity during the day.

With treatment, many people notice:

- Clearer thinking
- Better memory recall
- Improved focus at work
- Less "foggy" feeling during conversations
- Faster reaction time

These changes often feel small at first but become noticeable when you compare how you function now to how you felt before treatment.

Mood Often Stabilizes

Poor sleep stresses the nervous system.

Repeated oxygen drops trigger stress hormones that can increase irritability, anxiety, and emotional swings.

As sleep improves, many people notice:

- Less irritability
- Better patience
- More emotional steadiness
- Fewer morning mood crashes

Sleep doesn't fix everything, but it removes a constant biological stressor that was quietly affecting how you felt every day.

Your Body Gets a Break From Nightly Stress

Sleep apnea keeps the body in a cycle of nighttime emergency signals.

Each breathing pause triggers a surge in heart rate and blood pressure. Over time, this puts strain on the cardiovascular system and metabolism.

Consistent treatment can help:

- Lower nighttime blood pressure
- Reduce cardiovascular strain
- Improve insulin sensitivity
- Support healthier hormone regulation

These changes aren't always something you *feel* immediately, but they matter long term.

Snoring Often Improves - Which Helps Everyone in the Room

For people who share a bed or room, this may be one of the most noticeable changes.

Snoring often decreases dramatically once the airway stays open.
Breathing pauses stop.
Sleep becomes quieter and more stable.

For many couples, treating sleep apnea improves sleep for both people, not just the one using therapy.

You May Not Realize How Bad You Felt Before

One of the most common things people say after consistent treatment is: *"I didn't realize how tired I was until I wasn't."*

Sleep deprivation becomes normal when it's been happening long enough.
You adjust to functioning at half capacity.

When sleep improves, it doesn't just feel better, it often resets your sense of what normal energy actually is.

Change Takes Consistency

These improvements don't happen from using treatment once or twice. They build from consistent use over time.

Think of sleep recovery like rebuilding strength after an injury. One good night helps. Repeated good nights create real change. Consistency matters more than perfection.

What Comes Next

Once treatment is working and sleep improves, CPAP or other therapy often shifts from something you *have* to use… to something you rely on.

At that stage, people start thinking about practical life questions:

- How do I clean this properly?
- How do I travel with it?
- How do I maintain it long term?
- What actually matters and what's overkill?

That's where the final practical chapter comes in.

Chapter Thirteen

Living With CPAP: Cleaning, Travel, and Real-Life Maintenance

Once CPAP becomes part of your routine, the questions shift from “Can I tolerate this?” to “How do I live with this long term?”

Most of this is simpler than people expect. CPAP maintenance is not complicated, but a few habits make a big difference in comfort, hygiene, and equipment life.

This chapter focuses on the practical side of using CPAP in real life.

Cleaning Without Overcomplicating It

You do not need an elaborate system to keep CPAP equipment clean.

The goal is simply to prevent buildup of oils, moisture, and bacteria. The parts that need regular attention are:

Mask cushion
Tubing
Humidifier chamber

A simple routine works well for most people.

Wash the mask cushion with mild soap and warm water several times a week, or daily if your skin is oily or sensitive. This helps the seal stay effective and prevents irritation.

Rinse the humidifier chamber and let it air dry. Use distilled water if recommended by your provider or manufacturer.

Tubing usually only needs a wash once a week unless you notice odor, moisture buildup, or irritation.

You do not need special cleaners or machines. Mild soap, warm water, and air drying are usually enough. Consistency matters more than perfection.

Replacing Parts Before They Cause Problems

CPAP equipment does wear out over time.

Mask cushions soften, tubing stiffens, filters clog, and straps stretch. When this happens, comfort drops and leaks increase.

Many people struggle with CPAP simply because worn parts were never replaced.

General replacement timing varies, but common patterns include:

Mask cushions every few months
Filters monthly or as needed
Tubing every few months if it becomes stiff or discolored
Headgear when it stops holding fit properly

Insurance plans often cover replacement supplies on a schedule. Even if they do not, replacing worn parts usually costs far less than replacing a whole machine or quitting therapy.

If CPAP suddenly feels harder than it used to, worn equipment is often the reason.

Traveling With CPAP

Traveling with CPAP is easier than most people expect.

CPAP machines are considered medical devices, so airlines allow them as a separate carry item. They do not count toward your baggage limit. You do not need to check them unless you want to.

For air travel:

Carry the machine with you, not in checked luggage. Keep it in its travel case. Security screening is routine and common.

If you travel frequently, you may want:

A smaller travel CPAP model
A universal plug adapter for international travel
A backup extension cord in case outlets are far from the bed

Most hotels have no issue with CPAP use. If distilled water is needed, many hotels will provide it on request, or you can buy it locally. Travel does not have to interrupt therapy.

Keeping It Simple at Home

At home, small setup choices can make CPAP easier to live with.

Placing the machine slightly lower than your head can help reduce condensation in the tubing.

Using a hose holder or routing the tubing above the pillow can reduce pulling or tangling during the night.

Keeping supplies in one consistent place makes maintenance easier and reduces the chance of skipping cleaning or replacement.

CPAP works best when it becomes routine rather than something you constantly think about.

When Problems Show Up Later

Even after months of success, issues can still come up.

You might notice:

New mask leaks
Dryness returning
Pressure feeling different
Sleep changes due to weight or health shifts

This does not mean CPAP stopped working. It usually means something needs adjusting.

Most problems are solved by:

Replacing worn parts
Adjusting humidity
Checking mask fit
Talking with your provider about settings

CPAP is not a set-it-and-forget-it system forever. It is something you check in on occasionally, like any long-term health tool.

Living With CPAP Is Usually Easier Than People Expect

At the beginning, CPAP can feel like a big change.

Over time, most people stop noticing it much at all.

It becomes part of the nighttime routine, like brushing your teeth or setting an alarm. The focus shifts from the equipment to how you feel during the day.

Better sleep tends to make the maintenance feel worth it.

What Comes Next

At this point, you understand what sleep apnea is, how it is diagnosed, what treatment options exist, and what living with therapy actually looks like.

That leaves one final piece. What does all of this mean for your life going forward?

The last chapter pulls everything together and focuses on the bigger picture of sleep, health, and long-term change.

Chapter Fourteen

The Bigger Picture of Sleep and Health

By the time someone reaches this point, they usually understand sleep apnea in a way they did not before. They know it is not just snoring. They know it affects the body, the brain, and daily life. They know treatment is not always instant or perfect, but it is possible.

What matters most now is not the equipment or the diagnosis. It is what better sleep allows your life to become.

Sleep Is Not a Luxury

For a long time, many people treat sleep as optional.

They push through exhaustion.
They normalize brain fog.
They assume fatigue is just part of getting older or being busy.

But sleep is not downtime. It is active repair.

During sleep, the body regulates hormones, resets the nervous system, stabilizes metabolism, and supports brain function. When sleep is disrupted night after night, those systems never fully reset.

Treating sleep apnea is not about chasing perfect rest. It is about removing a barrier that has been quietly wearing your body down.

Treatment Is About Function, Not Perfection

Some nights will still be restless. Some nights equipment may feel annoying. Some nights life gets in the way.

That does not mean treatment failed.

Sleep improvement is about overall patterns, not flawless nights. If breathing is more stable most nights, the body has a chance to recover and protect itself long term.

Progress matters more than perfection.

What Better Sleep Often Changes

When sleep improves, people often notice changes they did not expect.

They may have more patience during the day. They may think more clearly at work.

They may have steadier moods. They may find it easier to stay awake during conversations, drives, or evening routines.

These shifts are not dramatic in a single moment. They build quietly over time.

Better sleep does not solve every problem in life. But it removes one of the biggest hidden stressors many people carry.

This Is Not About the Machine

For some people, treatment involves CPAP. For others, it may involve dental therapy, positional changes, or medical treatment.

The method matters less than the outcome.

The goal is simple: stable breathing during sleep so your body can finally rest the way it was meant to.

When that happens consistently, the benefits extend far beyond the night.

A Final Thought

If you were diagnosed recently, this may still feel new or uncertain.

If you have been living with sleep apnea for years, you may already know how much difference treatment can make.

Either way, understanding what is happening during sleep gives you something powerful.

It gives you the ability to take control of your health in a way many people never realize they need.

Sleep is not just about getting through the night. It shapes how you think, feel, and function every day that follows.

Taking care of your sleep is one of the most practical ways to take care of your life.

Authors Reflection

When I was first diagnosed with sleep apnea, I was told a lot of useful information by my doctor. The problem was that once I left the appointment, I could not find all of that information in one place.

Most of what I found online felt scattered, overly technical, or tied to selling a product, a machine, or a specific treatment. What I needed was something practical. Something that explained what was happening in plain language and what real life with treatment actually looks like.

That is why this book exists.

I did not see dramatic results overnight. It took months before I could look back and realize things had changed. At first the progress was small. A little less exhaustion. A little more focus. Fewer days where I felt like I could fall asleep sitting up.

Over time, those small steps added up.

I still wish I could roll out of bed the way I used to and feel instantly ready for the day. That part has not magically returned. But the trade-off is that I no longer feel like I need a nap just to get through the afternoon. My energy is steadier, and the fog that used to follow me around is not nearly as constant.

That matters.

If you are early in the process, it may not feel life-changing yet. That is normal. Most improvements show up gradually, not dramatically. The important part is consistency and giving your body time to adjust.

This book is not meant to replace medical advice, and it is not meant to push one specific treatment. It is simply a guide to help you understand what sleep apnea is, what treatment can look like, and what real progress often feels like.

If it helps you feel less confused, less overwhelmed, or more prepared for what comes next, then it has done its job.

T.L.Everheart

The information in this book is based on established sleep medicine research, clinical guidelines, and patient education resources. The references below include some of the major sources used in preparing this guide.

References

American Academy of Sleep Medicine. *Clinical Practice Guideline for Diagnostic Testing for Adult Obstructive Sleep Apnea.* Journal of Clinical Sleep Medicine.

American Academy of Sleep Medicine. *Clinical Guidelines for the Evaluation, Management, and Long-Term Care of Obstructive Sleep Apnea in Adults.*

National Heart, Lung, and Blood Institute. *Sleep Apnea.* U.S. Department of Health and Human Services.

Centers for Disease Control and Prevention. *Sleep and Sleep Disorders.*

National Sleep Foundation. *Sleep Apnea Information and Treatment Resources.*

Mayo Clinic. *Obstructive Sleep Apnea – Symptoms and Causes.*
Mayo Clinic. *Sleep Apnea – Diagnosis and Treatment.*

Cleveland Clinic. *Sleep Apnea: Overview, Diagnosis, and Treatment.*

Johns Hopkins Medicine. *Sleep Apnea and Snoring Information.*

Kryger, Meir H., Roth, Thomas, and Dement, William C. *Principles and Practice of Sleep Medicine.* Elsevier.

Weaver, T. E., and Grunstein, R. R. *Adherence to Continuous Positive Airway Pressure Therapy.* Proceedings of the American Thoracic Society.

Patil, S. P., et al. *Treatment of Adult Obstructive Sleep Apnea with Positive Airway Pressure: An American Academy of Sleep Medicine Clinical Practice Guideline.*

---

www.ingramcontent.com/pod-product-compliance
Lightning Source LLC
LaVergne TN
LVHW022231200926
848481LV00006B/2222
9798295705311